MW00354953

Surgical Knots
and
Suturing Techniques
Second Edition
Includes Basic Sterile Technique

F. D. Giddings

Giddings Studio Publishing

Fort Collins Colorado

2002

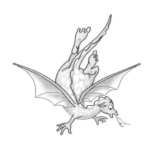

Printed in the United States of America

Giddings Studio Publishing
5913 Greenridge Circle
Fort Collins, Colorado 80525
Phone: 970-226-8587 Fax: 970-204-0543
e-mail: fdgid@lamar.colostate.edu

Library of Congress Control Number: 2002094245
Library of Congress Card Catalog Number: 97-93710

ISBN 978-1-889326-01-6

The second edition of Surgical Knots and Suturing Techniques follows the first after 5 years. The first edition included the techniques of knot tying as its primary content. Suture materials, surgical needles and the instruments used for knot tying and a section illustrating some common suture patterns made up the rest of the content.

This edition is intended for medical students, physician assistants, nurse practitioners, emergency medical technicians, surgical assistants, animal research specialists and the important but rarely addressed community of food animal producers. Important information for cleaning, sterilizing and preparing the surgical field in addition to closing acute wounds and incisions is included. Much of this information was previously available in *The Pocket Manual of Basic Surgical Skills*, Mosby, 1986. This book is no longer in print.

Professional medical and paramedical curricula include extensive training in aseptic and sterile technique as well as educating students in wound management. Animal science curricula educate the potential livestock producer in management procedures but leaves the problems involving the health of the animals to the veterinary profession. There are occasions, however, when stock producers are confronted with problems needing immediate attention. The procedures included in this book can be helpful in preparing those individuals for such crises.

Learning surgical knot tying and suturing techniques is challenging and much practice is required to develop proficiency. This book is a guide explaining and demonstrating the principle maneuvers of surgical knot tying along with a step-by-step description of each maneuver. The drawings make each step of knot tying understandable and easy to learn.

The necessary materials are available through medical school facilities and veterinary supply stores. Those veterinary supply stores serving the livestock producers are inclined to stock more of the supplies suggested in this book. Stores serving fewer food animal producers will stock fewer supplies. Stockmen needing supplies for emergency treatment of domestic animals should ask their veterinarians for materials and instruction.

Consultation with authors of the books I have illustrated for human and veterinary medicine over the past thirty five years is the primary source for the information contained in this book.

F. D. Giddings, AMI
Medical Illustrator Emeritus
College of Veterinary Medicine and Biomedical Sciences
Colorado State University, Fort Collins, Colorado

Contents

Describing surgical knot tying requires precise terminology. Terms of position and direction applied to the hands must be clear. The hand will be referred to as it appears in the anatomical position -- Standing in erect posture with the feet together, the arms hanging at the sides with the thumbs pointing away from the body.[4]

The median plane divides the body vertically into right and left halves. The terms *medial* and *lateral* refer to structures nearer to or farther away from the median plane.

The terms *proximal* and *distal* indicate a direction toward or away from the attached end of a limb, the origin of a structure or the center of the body.

The terms *palmar* and *dorsal* refer to the front and back of the hand.

The two figures below illustrate the terminology discussed here.

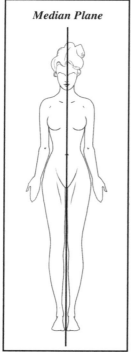

Anatomical Position

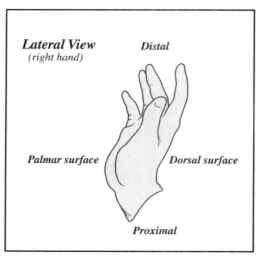

Lateral View of Right Hand

Terms describing actions of finger, thumb and wrist joints are explained in the following lateral view of the left hand. The terms *flexion, extension, pronation* and *supination are illustrated.*

F ... Flexion
E ... Extension
P ... Pronation
S ... Supination

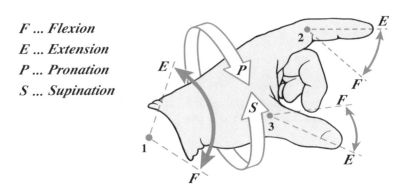

Flexion is to bend a joint and *extension* is to straighten a joint. In this illustration, three joints are used for demonstration:
   1.   Radiocarpal joint of the wrist
   2.   First interphalangeal joint of the index finger
   3.   Metacarpophalangeal joint of the thumb

The large dot indicates the pivot point for each extended or flexed joint. The gray arrows indicate flexion and extension.

Pronation is rotation of the thumb toward the body midline and *supination* is rotation of the thumb away from the body midline. The white arrow indicates pronation and supination.

Knots/Throws

When a surgeon refers to the number of "knots" used, the reference is to the number of half-knots or throws, not the number of completed knots. A half-knot or throw is a complete twist of two strands. A complete knot consists of two throws and is sometimes referred to as two knots.[1]

Three knots are commonly used in surgery:
- **Square Knot**
- **Surgeons' Knot**
- **Granny Knot (Slip Knot)**

The *square knot* is the most commonly used knot in surgery. It is tied by crossing the right strand over the left strand in the first throw followed by the left strand over the right in the second throw (*right-over-left, left-over-right*). If the square knot is started by crossing the left strand over the right, it must be finished by crossing the right strand over the left. When this sequence of throws or half-knots is performed, the square knot will not slip.

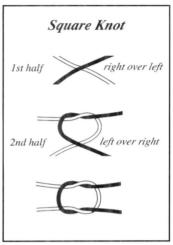

Square Knot

1st half — *right over left*

2nd half — *left over right*

The *surgeons' knot* is a square knot which contains a double twist in the first throw. The double twist makes the first throw of the knot less likely to slip while the second throw is being tied.

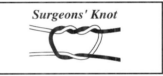

Surgeons' Knot

The *granny knot* is a "pseudosquare knot". The strands of the second throw cross in the same sequence as the strands of the first throw (*right-over-left, right-over-left*). The result is a *slip knot* which is useful when the finished knot must be "slipped" down to tighten. Its holding qualities are not good and it should be backed up with a square knot.

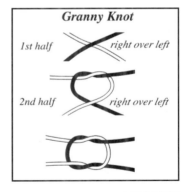

Granny Knot

1st half — *right over left*

2nd half — *right over left*

Pulling one strand of a granny knot will demonstrate how the knot transforms into a slip knot.[1]

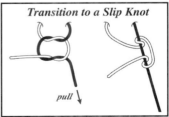

Transition to a Slip Knot

pull

Surgical Knots and Suturing Techniques is divided into two sections:
>   Section I,   Techniques and Materials for Tying Surgical Knots
>   Section II,   Suture Hardware, Suturing Methods, Suture Patterns,
>   Basic Sterile Technique.

Traditionally, surgical knots have been described as *Two-Handed* and *One-Handed*. However, in both styles, there is a *"tying hand"* and a *"non-tying hand"*. The non-tying hand simply manipulates the free end of the suture. The tying hand is usually the non-dominant hand. A right handed individual would use the left hand as the tying hand.[1] This book shows the left hand tying the knots. To view the drawings with the right hand tying, place this book in front of a mirror.

The *two-handed tie* described in this book may be easier to tie for the beginning student because it uses less finger action and more arm and wrist action.

Three styles of *one-handed throws* are described. The first half-knot will produce a right-over-left throw. The second, a left-over-right throw and the third a right-over-left. Try all of the one-handed styles, then select the sequence you like best making sure it will form a square knot.

To practice the knots, punch two holes one centimeter apart and one centimeter from the edge of a 5" x 7" note card. Pass a piece of string 30 inches long through one hole and out the other resulting in two tying ends. Secure the card so the edge with the holes and string face you. Darken one of the strands with a felt tip pen to match the black and white strands seen in the illustrations in this handbook.

The suture material in the knot tying directions has been illustrated in a size large enough to permit visualization of the short (black) and long (white) strands. Actual suture material, for most closures, is much smaller and would look like fine thread.

The basis for the ability to inject drugs, treat wounds and the entire field of operative surgery is a group of techniques known as *aseptic* or *sterile* technique. The difference between aseptic and sterile technique is subtle. *Aseptic* refers to the complete absence of living microorganisms brought about by physical means such as autoclaving or gamma irradiation. *Sterile* also refers to the complete absence of living microorganisms but the state may be produced using disinfectants (chemical agents)[1]. Disinfectant solutions available without prescription are used in the sterile techniques of this book.

Techniques and Materials for Tying
Surgical Knots

First Throw

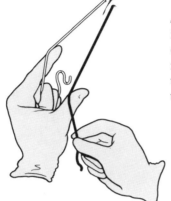

Step 1. Hold the short suture (black) in the right hand. The long suture (white) is held under the left ring and middle fingers. Keeping the left thumb and index finger apart, place the sutures as shown.

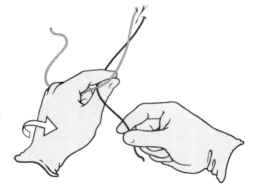

Step 2. Touch the left thumb and index finger. Pronate the left hand to form an opening between the sutures.

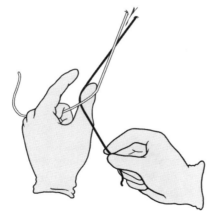

Step 3. Elevate the left thumb through the opening. Release the left index finger leaving the sutures around the thumb.

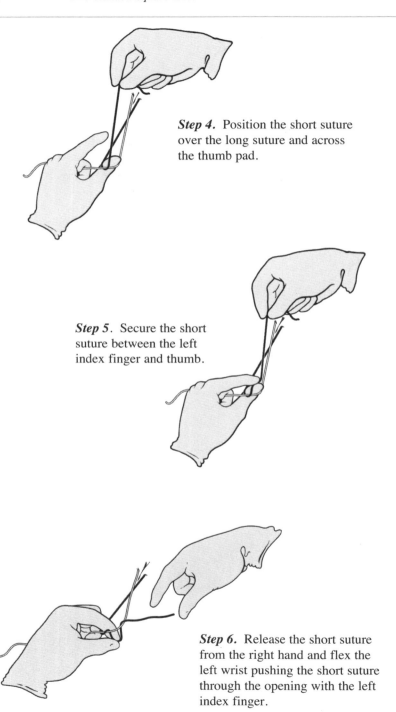

Step 4. Position the short suture over the long suture and across the thumb pad.

Step 5. Secure the short suture between the left index finger and thumb.

Step 6. Release the short suture from the right hand and flex the left wrist pushing the short suture through the opening with the left index finger.

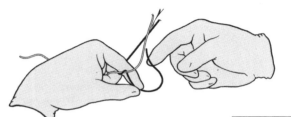

Step 7. When the short suture has passed completely through the opening, it is again picked up with the right hand.*

> *When tying a surgeons' knot, make a double twist before tightening the first throw.*

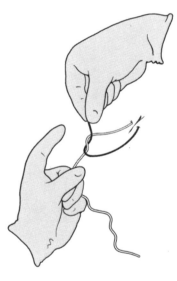

Step 8. Move the right hand distally and flex the wrist. Extend the left wrist. The hands are now in position to tighten the throw.

Step 9. Use the left index finger to tighten the throw. This action also facilitates tightening throws in deep cavities. The inset shows the suture lying flat to prevent slipping of the completed throw.

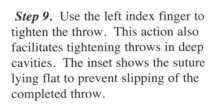

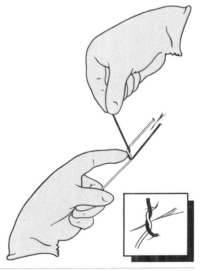

Second Throw

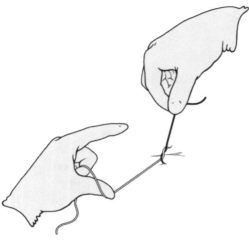

Step 10. Withdraw the left index finger. Keep holding the long suture under the left middle and ring fingers. Begin the second throw by securing the long suture with the left thumb.

Step 11. Bring the short suture across the long suture between the left thumb and middle finger. Take care not to pull the suture strands too tight to avoid the possibility of dislodging the first throw.

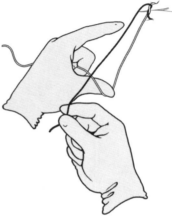

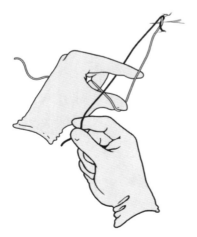

Step 12. The left index finger will pass over the short suture and into the newly formed opening between the short and long suture strands.

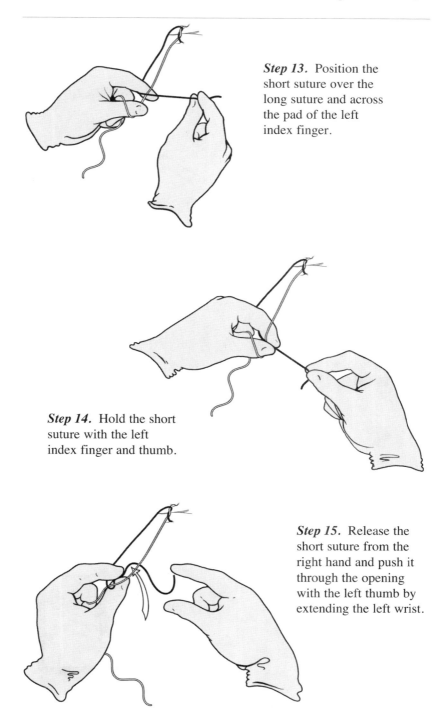

Step 13. Position the short suture over the long suture and across the pad of the left index finger.

Step 14. Hold the short suture with the left index finger and thumb.

Step 15. Release the short suture from the right hand and push it through the opening with the left thumb by extending the left wrist.

Step 16. Pronate the right hand and
move it toward you while holding
the end of the short suture with the
thumb and index finger. This action
will remove suture twisting and
allow the knot to lie flat.

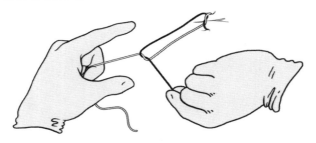

Step 17. To complete the knot,
pronate the left hand pushing the
throw flat with the left index finger.
The inset shows the finished knot
before it is drawn tight.

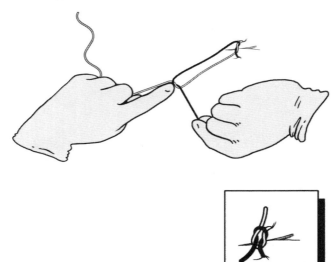

Three techniques performing one-handed throws are presented in this section. Technique I followed by Technique II will produce a square knot. Technique III followed by Technique II will also produce a square knot. Memorize either combination after experimenting with each sequence.

Technique I

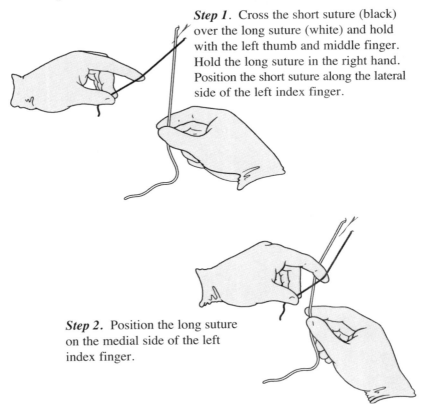

Step 1. Cross the short suture (black) over the long suture (white) and hold with the left thumb and middle finger. Hold the long suture in the right hand. Position the short suture along the lateral side of the left index finger.

Step 2. Position the long suture on the medial side of the left index finger.

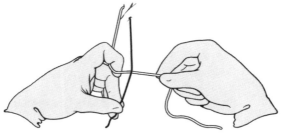

Step 3. Flex the left index finger engaging the long suture on its palmar side.

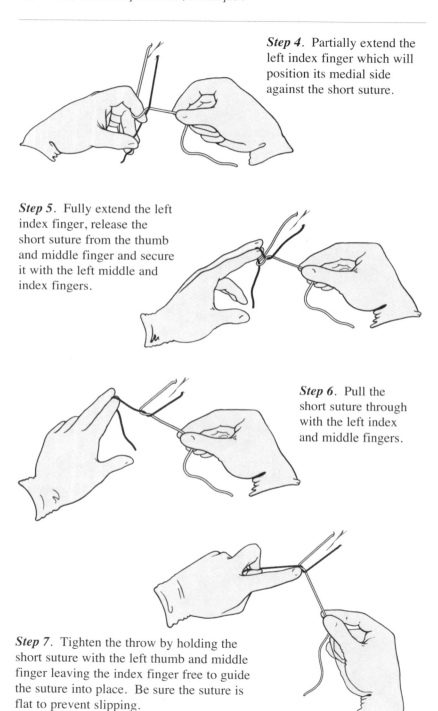

Step 4. Partially extend the left index finger which will position its medial side against the short suture.

Step 5. Fully extend the left index finger, release the short suture from the thumb and middle finger and secure it with the left middle and index fingers.

Step 6. Pull the short suture through with the left index and middle fingers.

Step 7. Tighten the throw by holding the short suture with the left thumb and middle finger leaving the index finger free to guide the suture into place. Be sure the suture is flat to prevent slipping.

Technique II

Step 1. With the palm of the left hand facing up, hold the short suture between the thumb and index finger having the suture pass across the palmar surface of the other three fingers.

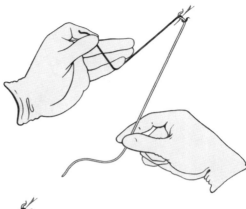

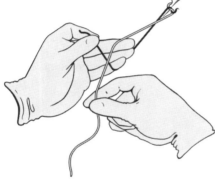

Step 2. Position the long suture on the lateral side of the left middle finger then across the short suture between the ring and little fingers.

Step 3. Flex the left middle finger to engage the long suture.

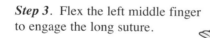

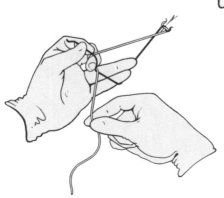

Step 4. Continue flexing the left middle finger to engage the short suture on its dorsal surface.

Step 5. Extend the left middle finger and secure the short suture between it and the left ring finger. Release the short suture from the left thumb and index finger.

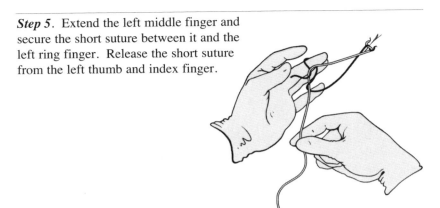

Step 6. The short suture is pulled through. The throw will appear to be twisted and backward but the next step will alleviate this problem.

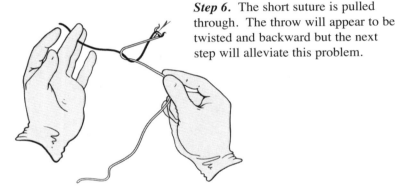

Step 7. Cross the left hand distal to the right hand. Hold the long suture between the right thumb and middle finger leaving the index finger free to guide the throw down completing the knot.

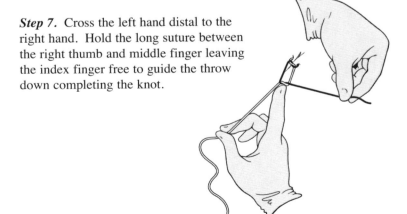

Technique III

Step 1. Cross the short suture (black) over the long suture (white) and hold with the left thumb and index finger. Hold the long suture in the right hand. Face the left palm up and place the long suture on the medial side of the left ring finger.

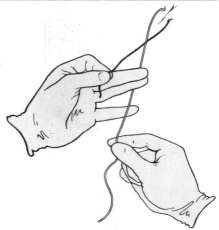

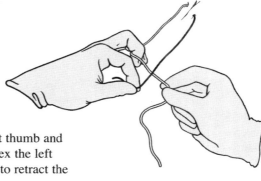

Step 2. Pronate the left hand securing the long suture under the middle and ring fingers. The sutures cross a finger width distal to the left index finger.

Step 3. Keeping the left thumb and index finger together, flex the left middle and ring fingers to retract the long suture.

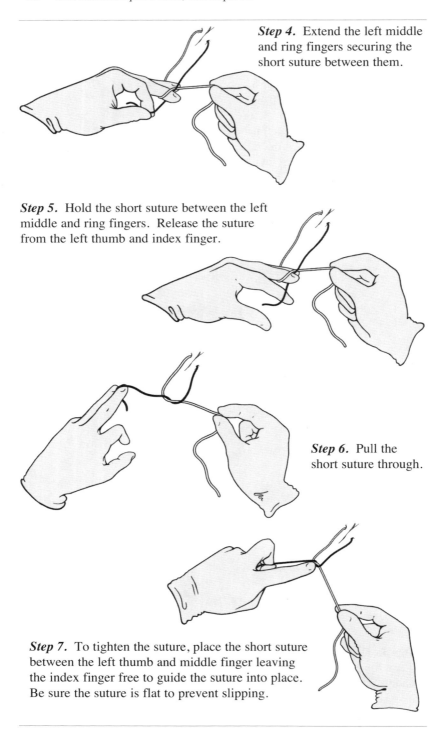

Step 4. Extend the left middle and ring fingers securing the short suture between them.

Step 5. Hold the short suture between the left middle and ring fingers. Release the suture from the left thumb and index finger.

Step 6. Pull the short suture through.

Step 7. To tighten the suture, place the short suture between the left thumb and middle finger leaving the index finger free to guide the suture into place. Be sure the suture is flat to prevent slipping.

First Throw

Step 1. With the needle holder in the
right hand, place the needle through
the tissue. Pull the suture through
leaving a 2 cm end.

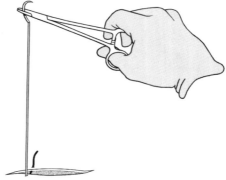

Step 2. Release the needle from the holder and grasp it
with the left hand. Position the needle holder against
the far side of the suture near its midpoint.

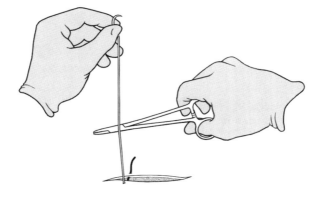

Step 3. With the left hand, wrap the suture around the needle holder once for a square knot.*

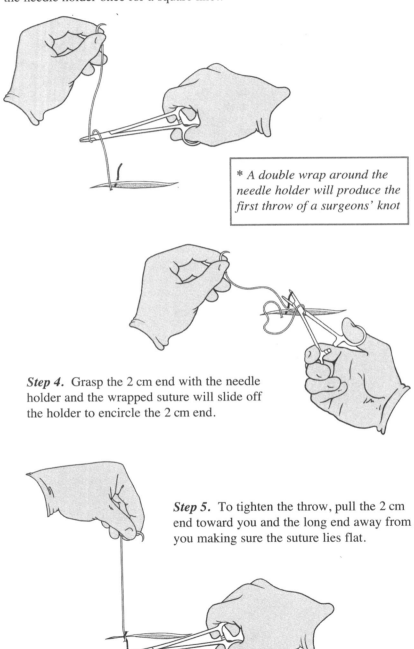

> * *A double wrap around the needle holder will produce the first throw of a surgeons' knot*

Step 4. Grasp the 2 cm end with the needle holder and the wrapped suture will slide off the holder to encircle the 2 cm end.

Step 5. To tighten the throw, pull the 2 cm end toward you and the long end away from you making sure the suture lies flat.

Second Throw

Step 6. Release the 2 cm end from the needle holder. Position the needle holder against the near side of the suture and wrap the long end once around the needle holder with the left hand.

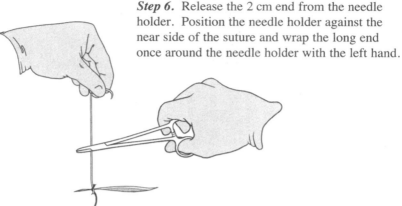

Step 7. Grasp the 2 cm end in the needle holder and pull it through the wrap.

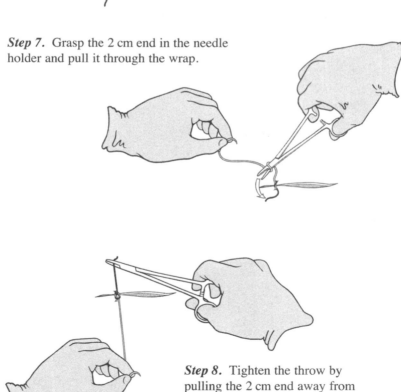

Step 8. Tighten the throw by pulling the 2 cm end away from you and the long end toward you.

The Miller's knot is tied over a clamp before being transferred to the pedicle. The knot can also be tied directly on the pedicle.

Step 1. Hold one end of the suture in the left hand under the middle, ring and little fingers. Control 8" of free suture with the right hand. Place the medial side of the left index finger on the clamp and loosely wrap the free end of the suture clockwise around the index finger and clamp.

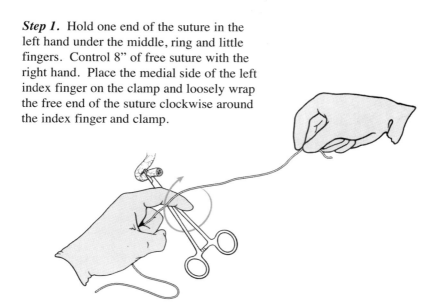

Step 2. Bring the left thumb and index finger together and extend the left wrist. This action will bring the thumb through the wrap.

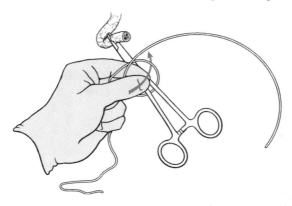

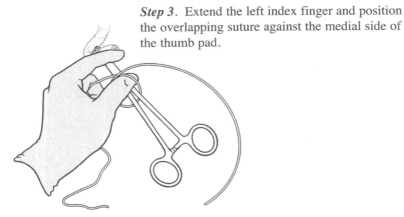

Step 3. Extend the left index finger and position the overlapping suture against the medial side of the thumb pad.

Step 4. Bring the tip of the left index finger in front of the 8" free suture, under the first wrap and again touch the left thumb. Flex the left wrist to facilitate this step.

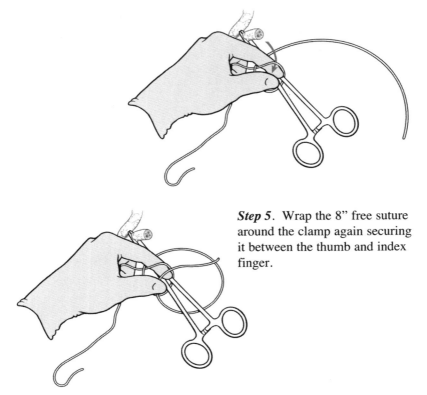

Step 5. Wrap the 8" free suture around the clamp again securing it between the thumb and index finger.

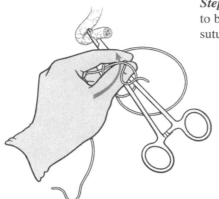

Step 6. Extend the left wrist to bring the free end of the suture through the wrap.

Step 7. Slide the knot off the end of the clamp onto the pedicle. To tighten the knot, pull evenly on both ends of the suture. The knot is secure and will compress the pedicle. The ligature will not loosen at this point.

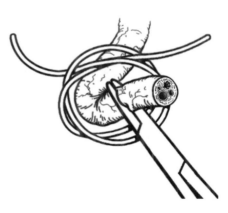

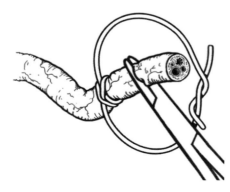

Step 8. Both suture ends should be taken 180° around the pedicle and secured with a simple square knot.

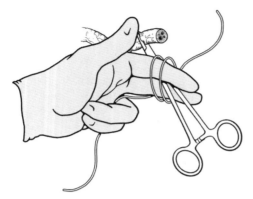

Step 1. Hold the suture under the ring and little fingers of the left hand while placing the clamp between the index and middle fingers. Make two loose counterclockwise wraps around the clamp and fingers.

Step 2. Touch the left thumb and index finger, extend the left wrist to bring them through the suture wraps.

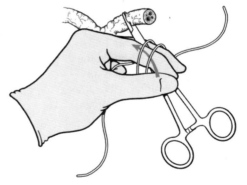

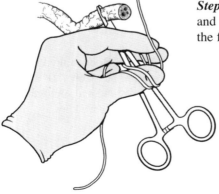

Step 3. Separate the thumb and index finger and place the free suture in their grip.

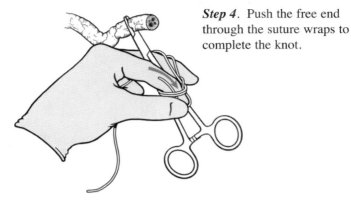

Step 4. Push the free end through the suture wraps to complete the knot.

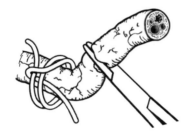

Step 5. Slide the knot off the holder and over the pedicle before tightening.

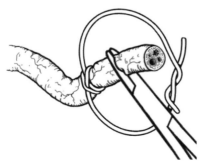

Step 6. Both suture ends should be taken 180° around the pedicle and secured with a simple square knot.

Section II

Suture Hardware
Suturing Methods
Suture Patterns
Basic Sterile Technique

Suture materials have two very important characteristics:
- Absorbable
- Nonabsorbable

Absorbable sutures, as their name implies, are absorbed by the body after several weeks. Gut has been the principal absorbable material but fine new synthetic materials are gaining popularity.

Absorbable sutures are made from the following materials:
- Absorbable surgical gut
  - Plain, the intestinal submucosa of sheep intestine or serosa of beef intestine.
  - Chromic, plain gut soaked in chromic acid salts.
- Polyglycolonate, (Maxon, USS/DG)
- Polybutester, (Novafil, Vascufil, USS/DG)
- Polyglactin 910 (Vicryl, Ethicon)
- Poliglecaprone 25 (Monocryl, Ethicon) [5]
- PDS II (Polydioxanone, Ethicon) [5]

Nonabsorbable sutures are used for skin and fascial closure as well as vessel ligation. They are supplied in four basic types:
- Natural fibers of cotton and silk
- Braided synthetics
- Monofilament synthetics
- Stainless steel

Early surgeons used the natural fibers of cotton and silk for suturing. They are easy to handle, however, cotton will hold secure with fewer throws. Silk is less likely to cause infection as it lacks the capillarity of cotton and will tie securely with 3 half-knots or throws. Silk is manufactured in twisted and braided forms.[1,2]

Braided synthetics are manufactured in nylon and other polymers listed above. The braided synthetics are less reactive than silk but require 5-6 throws for knot security leaving more suture material in the wound.[2]

Monofilament synthetic sutures made of nylon, polybutester and polypropylene are the most inert. Nylon and polypropylene are difficult to handle and tie and the knots are not steadfast but polybutester (Novafil) handles and ties well. Because synthetics are the most inert, they do not tend to harbor bacteria making them more desirable for infected wounds.[2]

Steel sutures are made of stainless steel available as monofilament and braided suture. Steel wire sutures are not easily placed in tissue and they are extremely difficult to tie but when they are used the knot security is excellent. Large sizes are too cumbersome to tie and must be twisted. Steel wire is advantageous when suturing bone as the desired degree of tension can be regulated by twisting the wire.

Suture material is sized by two methods:
- United States Pharmacopeia (USP)
- Metric.

USP sizes range from 7-0 the largest size, to 14-0 the smallest. Metric sizing expresses the suture diameter in tenths of a millimeter. A USP size 7-0 is equivalent to a metric 41 gauge (4.1 mm). USP suture sizes for skin and subcutis are 4-0 to 3-0, for fascia and tendon 3-0 to 0, for vessel ligatures 4-0 to 2-0 and for vessel and nerve sutures 6-0 to 5-0.[2]

Several factors enter into suture material selection. Absorbable sutures are used when continued strength is not important or when infection makes it desirable for the suture to be absorbed. Absorbable sutures are used for subcutaneous tissues and for mucosal layers of the intestine.[2]

Nonabsorbable suture is used when continued strength is important, when the sutures are to be removed after healing and when minimal tissue reaction is important. Nonabsorbable sutures are used for skin and fascial closure and for small vessel ligation.[2]

Hundreds of needle types are manufactured but most surgeons are familiar with only a few dozen.[1] All needles have four characteristics:
- Needle to suture attachment
- Point and cross section
- Shape of needle shaft
- Size

Needle to suture attachment is accomplished with an eye or a swaged attachment accomplished during the manufacturing process.

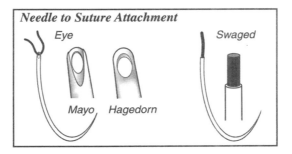

Needle to Suture Attachment

Eye Swaged

Mayo Hagedorn

Needles with eyes must be 3x to 4x as thick as the suture and leave large holes in the tissue. This is not a problem in skin and fascia but is not acceptable when suturing bowel or blood vessels. Swaged needles are only slightly larger in diameter than the suture and leave much smaller holes in the tissue.[1]

Needle point and cross section are determined by the tissue being sutured. *Tapered needles*, round in cross section, are used for soft tissue (gastrointestinal, urinary bladder) and fascia. Cutting needles are used for more dense tissues like skin and tendon. *Conventional cutting needles* are three sided with the cutting apex of the triangle directed toward the center of a curved needle. The needle cuts in the direction of the suture pull and it

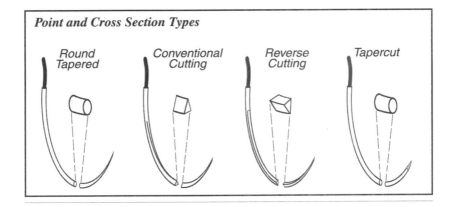

Point and Cross Section Types

Round Tapered   Conventional Cutting   Reverse Cutting   Tapercut can be curved or straight. *Reverse cutting needles* place a cut away from the pull of the suture and are used in the skin. Vascular surgery requires fine needles sharp enough to penetrate synthetic vascular graft material but not so sharp that they damage delicate blood vessel walls.[1] *Tapercut needles* are used for this purpose as they readily penetrate the graft material while passing through the tissue without cutting the suture path.

Selection of the needle shape is determined in part by the type, depth and accessibility of the tissue. Straight needles are usually hand held and are used on surface wounds. Curved needles are held with needle holders and are used for small surface wounds and wounds deep in the body cavity.[2]

The needle shafts are curved, half curved and straight.

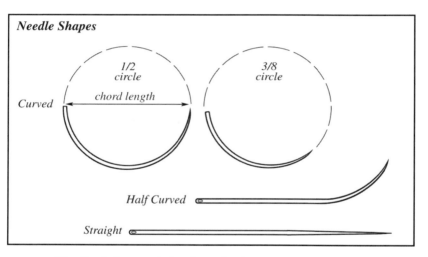

Needle Shapes

Curved — 1/2 circle — chord length — 3/8 circle

Half Curved

Straight

The final characteristic of needles is size. The size of a needle is equal to the needle chord length measured across the circle diameter rather than along its curve. A 1/2 circle needle could be the same size as a 3/8 circle needle but the 1/2 circle needle is 25% longer. A needle should be large enough to permit rapid, accurate and precise suturing.[2]

Specific choices in the selection of suture materials, needle style and size can only be determined by experience. The scope of this book is to teach the basics of suturing. More advanced schooling in the individual specialties along with experience will lead to practical selections.

The placement of sutures to close wounds is accomplished in most cases with the use of needle holders and tissue forceps. Needle holders are similar to hemostatic forceps, however, their tips are shorter and heavier with jaws grooved with a pattern conducive to holding a needle securely.[1]

Three grasping techniques are employed:

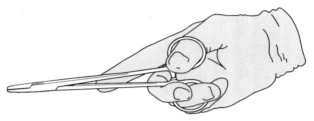

Thumb and third finger grip facilitates rapid grasping and releasing.

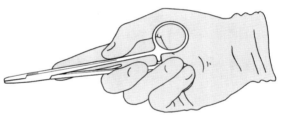

Palm grip allows greater force for insertion of the needle.

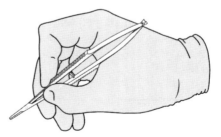

Pencil grip offers maximum control of fine needles.[2]

Tissue forceps are called thumb forceps and are designed to hold and immobilize tissue during the placement of sutures. *Toothed* thumb forceps are used to grasp subcutaneous tissue, fat, muscle and skin for closure. More delicate tissues of the viscera and blood vessels are held with *smooth* thumb forceps.[1]

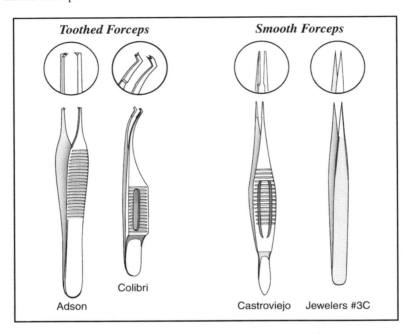

Toothed Forceps   **Smooth Forceps**

Colibri

Adson   Castroviejo   Jewelers #3C

In most surgical situations needle holders grasp the needle with its axis perpendicular to the long axis of the needle holder,[2] however, when a suture must be placed in a deep hole, the needle is placed in the holder at a steep angle. A needle grasped near the tip applies greater force to pene-trate dense tissues. Grasp the needle near its midpoint for general purpose suturing and near the suture end to achieve finest control when suturing delicate tissues.[2]

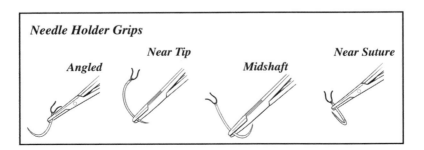

Needle Holder Grips

Near Tip   *Near Suture*

Angled   *Midshaft*

Guidelines for tying sutures and ligatures:

- The size of the suture need only be large enough to provide adequate strength for the tissues being sutured.[3]

- Pass the needle through the tissue in a direction towards you.[6]

- Provide even tension to both strands of each throw to form comfortably secure knots. Firmly approximating tissues may cause too much tension caused by edema the next day.[3]

- Approximate all tissues as a deep wound is closed to avoid spaces within the tissues. Spaces can increase the likelihood of infection.[3]

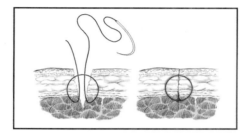

- The distance of the needle puncture from the edge of the wound should be equal to the depth of the layer of tissue being sutured and include equal amounts of tissue on either side of the wound. Different amounts of tissue or different suture depths cause the skin edges to overlap. A distance of one fourth inch (0.5 cm) is good for strong tissue like skin. Delicate viscera, blood vessels and nerves require finer, closely approximated sutures.[2]

- Trim completed knots to minimize reaction to suture material. Free ends of cotton, silk and synthetic materials are trimmed to 3 mm. Trim the ends of absorbable materials to 6 mm.[2]

- Carry the throws down to the tissue with the tip of the index finger to prevent damaging the suture material. Damaged suture material weakens the knot.[2]

- Tie the minimum number of throws necessary to secure knots. Extra throws add bulk which increases foreign material tissue reaction.[2]

Suture patterns can be placed in two ways:
- Interrupted
- Continuous

An *interrupted* suture consists of single stitches placed in a row and each stitch has its own knot.

Continuous sutures begin with the initial knot and run continuously to the end of the wound before the finishing knot is tied.

Interrupted suture patterns offer the security that comes from each stitch having its own knot. The tension of each suture along the incision can be adjusted during execution of each stitch.

Speed is the major advantage of continuous suture patterns because all the stitches needed to close a wound can be finished with one knot. If the wound becomes infected, all stitches must be removed. Some continuous patterns allow tension adjustment at multiple points along the wound.[1]

When placing the needle, use an approach that permits comfortable use of instruments. The right handed surgeon can place the needle from right to left or top to bottom depending on the orientation of the wound.

Apply opposing forces to the knot "ears" that are equal in magnitude and in a plane parallel to that of the wound surface.[6]

Clamp only the free end of the suture during an instrument tie. Clamping the suture will damage and weaken the material.[6]

The following pages contain illustrations of suture patterns in three categories:
- Appositional sutures
- Tension sutures
- Inverting sutures

Over-and-Over

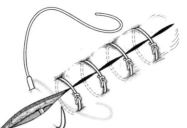

The *over-and-over* pattern on the left is *simple interrupted*. Each stitch is tied with a square knot.

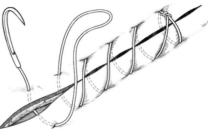

Over-and-over continuous is the pattern on the right. A square knot is used to finish the first stitch. The suture continues as a running stitch until the wound is closed.

Securing Continuous Suture Patterns

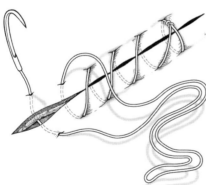

Secure the continuous suture during the placement of the last stitch. Leave a length of suture long enough to double back and serve as one tying strand of the final knot. Pull enough suture through the last stitch to make up the second tying strand. When each strand is the proper length, tie a square knot.

The first throw of the final knot is in progress at the right. Finish the knot with as many throws as the suture material and wound require.

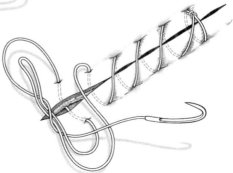

Intradermal or Subcuticular

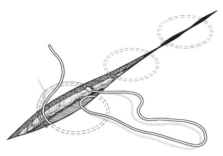

The continuous *intradermal* pattern, also called a *subcuticular* suture is placed as an interrupted pattern at the left. It is placed as continuous below. This is a cosmetic closure because it leaves no suture marks. For safety, it should be reinforced with "steri-strips".

To complete the continuous intradermal subcuticular suture, carry the needle through the apposing side of the wound and tie off using the directions for securing continuous patterns on page 33.

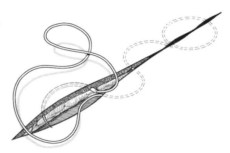

Locking Stitch (Ford Interlocking)

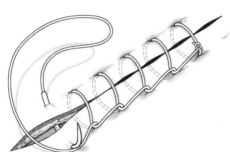

The *locking stitch*, or *Ford interlocking* stitch is a continuous pattern formed by placing the emerging needle so it passes over the suture from the preceding stitch. It is finished with the method shown on page 33.

This continuous pattern provides greater security than the simple continuous over-and-over pattern and suture tension can be adjusted with each stitch.

Interrupted Cruciate

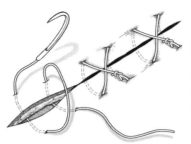

The *interrupted cruciate*, also called the *cross mattress* pattern, is stronger than the simple interrupted pattern. It is the easiest mattress suture to apply and the pattern resists tissue eversion.

Horizontal Mattress

The *horizontal mattress* suture is shown as an interrupted pattern on the left and continuous on the right. With the interrupted pattern the sutures lie parallel to the wound edges making each stitch equivalent to two simple interrupted stitches. Minor blood vessels along the wound edges are constrained by the horizontal sutures.

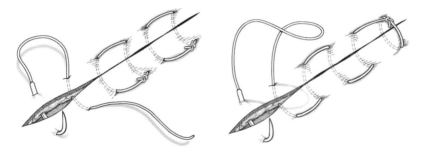

Vertical Mattress

The *vertical mattress* takes deep and superficial bites insignificantly constraining minor blood vessels while providing maximum suture strength.

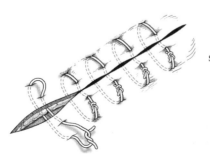

This enlarged view shows superficial and deep suture bites.

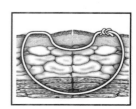

Inverting Sutures

Surgeries, like anastomosis of the stomach, require inversion of the wound edges. Simply apposing mucosa to mucosa will not provide a good seal. Serosa sutured to serosa will be secure if the suture material does not penetrate all layers of the stomach wall. Infection can follow needle paths from the interior to the outside of the stomach. A secure anastomosis of the stomach can be accomplished using two layers of sutures: an inverting suture through all stomach layers and an outer suture passing through only the serosa and muscularis.

Cushing

The *Cushing suture* pattern is a good primary closure of the stomach inverting the edges of the wall and apposing the serosal surfaces. The suture is continued completely around the circumference of the anastomosis and tied to the free end of the first stitch. This is shown in progress here. Absorbable suture is used.

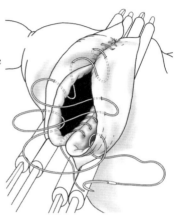

A secure anastomosis is accomplished with the Cushing pattern but it must be backed up with an outer suture such as the Lembert described below.

Lembert

The *Lembert suture* passes through the serosa, muscularis and a small part of the submucosa on each side of the previously placed Cushing. When it is tightened, the edges of the serosa are pulled together inverting the Cushing pattern. Lembert sutures can be interrupted or continuous. Finish continuous Lembert suture patterns with the method described on page 33.

The diagram at the right illustrates a section of anastomosed stomach with interrupted Lembert stitches placed over a Cushing pattern.

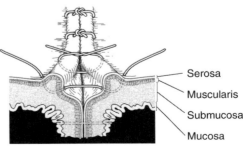

Serosa

Muscularis

Submucosa

Mucosa

Suture removal should be a painless procedure. The wound should be swabbed with an antiseptic and dried exudate removed. The knot or a loose end of the stitch is grasped with forceps providing gentle elevation of the stitch. The suture is cut with scissors or a number 11 scalpel blade where it enters the skin. The suture is withdrawn with the forceps. The forceps are holding the knot so it won't be drawn through the suture path causing contamination.[1]

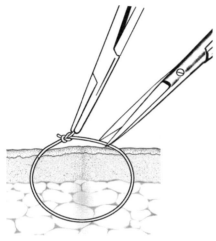

Snip the suture close to where it enters the skin.

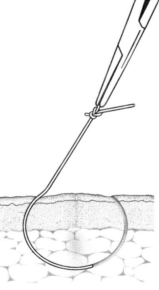

Pull with the forceps to complete the suture removal.

Infection is introduced into the body from outside. Infection can be avoided by seeing to it that any procedure involving the interruption of the skin is carried out in a sterile field, an area void of all living bacteria. The skin, all instruments and the hands of the surgeon must be cleaned and sterilized. Antimicrobial detergent soaps containing chlorhexidine gluconate (Hibiclens), hexachlorophene (pHisoHex), and iodophor (Betadine) are used for washing skin and hands. Sterile gloves should encase the surgeon's hands or the procedure must be done without the surgeon's hands touching the sterile field or the ends of the sterile instruments.[1]

Hand Preparation

Even when covered with sterile gloves, the surgeon's hands should be scrubbed. Iodophor, hexachlorophene and chlorhexidine gluconate are used for this purpose. The Betadine surgical prep brush packets are ideal.

The standard scrub technique requires first cleaning the nails. Any visible dirt should be removed with a nail file or plastic nail pick followed by vigorous brushing. A five minute scrub beginning with the fingers and thumbs then the hands and up the forearms to the elbows should follow.

Skin Preparation

The first step in wound care is to cleanse the wound and surrounding skin. Gross contaminants such as dirt or grease should be removed using one of the three detergent soaps listed above.

Wound Irrigation

The antimicrobial detergent soaps used for cleaning the skin are cytotoxic and should not be used for wound irrigation. Copius irrigation should be done using sterile saline solution applied with a sterile bulb syringe or a large sterile disposable syringe. Light scrubbing with a gloved hand can help remove gross debris. Care should be taken not to injure the tissue.[7]

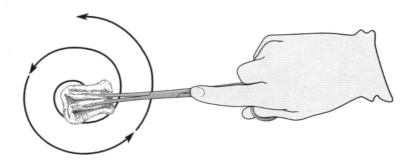

When the operative field is scrubbed, begin at the center and work outward unless the wound is contaminated. For contaminated wounds, cleanse the surrounding skin first and the wound last. The area prepared should be much larger than the operative field. The illustration on page 38 shows the preparation technique.

Debridement

Debridement is used to remove necrotic tissue or tissue containing gross contamination not removed by irrigation. If necessary, healthy tissue can be removed from the wound margins for better approximation of tissue layers.[7]

Iodine

Iodine is one of the oldest and most effective antiseptic solutions. Tincture of iodine is available through veterinary supply houses in a 7% solution in isopropyl alcohol. Iodine in this form can be mildly toxic and burn the skin. It is best to clean the skin with isopropyl alcohol immediately after use. Betadine is a compound in which iodine is combined with an organic molecule (iodophor). The iodine is released from the organic complex slowly enough to avoid burning but fast enough to kill bacteria. In the operating room the skin is first cleansed with detergent containing Betadine solution which is allowed to dry then painted with nondetergent Betadine which leaves a thin film of iodophor on the skin. For hand washing, disposable Betadine scrub sponges are available through veterinary supply houses.

Alcohol

Alcohol is used to prepare the skin prior to shots and venapuncture, however, it does not adequately kill bacteria. It is a good cleaning agent but not a good antiseptic.

Mercury

Mercury containing solutions have been used in the past in such forms as Mercurochrome and Merthiolate. Mercurochrome is ineffective as an antiseptic. While Merthiolate is more effective, it penetrates the skin poorly and does not kill spores.[1]

Iodophor

Iodophors are a group of compounds in which iodine is combined with an organic molecule.

Iodophor containing detergent will cause the bacterial count to drop markedly in the first minute. After five minutes the count will be minimal.

Sterilizing Instruments

Instruments are sterilized using steam autoclaving, ethylene oxide gas, cold sterilization and irradiation.

Steam autoclaving is used to prepare instruments and instrument packs. Metal instruments not wrapped require 15 minutes at a temperature of 120° C (250° F). Wrapped packets require 30 minutes. Steam will not penetrate the jaws of closed clamps or small caliber needles.

Ethylene oxide is a gas which sterilizes at temperatures of 50° to 60° C (120° to 150° F). It is used for instruments that are damaged by heat.

Cold sterilization, involves soaking instruments in germicidal solutions such as iodophor or formalin. Instruments should be soaked for at least 30 minutes then rinsed in a sterile water or saline solution before use.

Irradiation using high dose gamma irradiation from a cobalt source is used by the manufactures of medical devices.

• • •

To insure that all bacteria are excluded from the sterile field, these basic techniques must be followed in all invasive procedures.

References

1. Van Way C.W., Buerk C.A.: *Pocket Manual of Basic Surgical Skills*, The C.V. Mosby Company, St. Louis, 1986. (*out of print*)

2. Slatter D.: *Textbook of Small Animal Surgery*, 2nd Ed., W.B. Saunders Company, Philadelphia, 1993.

3. Nealon T.F.: *Fundamental Skills in Surgery*, W.B. Saunders Company, Philadelphia, 1971.

4. Gray H.: *Anatomy of the Human Body*, Lea & Febiger, Philadelphia, 1967.

5. *Ethicon Wound Closure Manual*, www.jnjgateway.com/home.jhtml, 2002.

6. *USS/DG Knot Tying Manual*, www.ussdgsutures.com, 2002

7. Doherty, G.M., et. al. *The Washington Manual of Surgery,* Little, Brown and Company, 1997.

8. Piermattei, D.L., *An Atlas of Surgical Approaches to the Bones and Joints of the Dog and Cat, 3rd edition*, 1993.

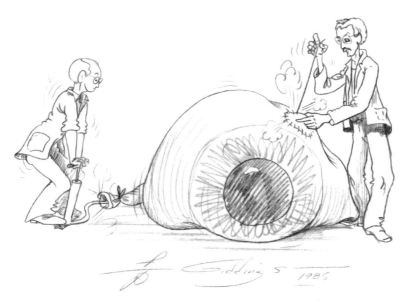

"Learning surgical knot tying and suturing techniques is challenging and much practice is required to develop proficiency."

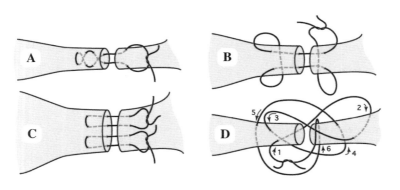

Tendon and ligament suture patterns. **A.** Modified Bunnell-Mayer used in small tendons cut close to the bone. **B.** Horizontal mattress used in large flat tendons. **C.** Locking loop (Kessler) creates very secure closure for tendon or ligament. **D.** Pulley suture used for small tendons or ligaments. Initial passes 1 and 2 placed near and far. Passes 3 and 4 are placed 120° from 1 and 2 and midway between near–far positions. Passes 5 and 6 are placed 120° from 3 and 4 in a far–near pattern.[8]